Table of Contents

Understanding and Managing Stomach Bloating After Eating

1. Introduction to Stomach Bloating

1.1. Definition and Causes of Stomach Bloating

2. Common Causes of Stomach Bloating After Eating

2.1. Overeating

2.2. Eating Too Quickly

2.3. Food Intolerances and Sensitivities

3. Gut Health and Stomach Bloating

3.1. Role of Gut Microbiota in Digestion

4. Dietary Strategies to Reduce Stomach Bloating

Understanding the Causes and Solutions for Post-Meal Bloating

1. Introduction to Post-Meal Bloating

Some people may take Beano-like tablets to prevent bloating due to vegetables, fruits, and whole grains containing fibers by breaking it into ink everyday doses whose packets are also steady for consumption over time. To get instant relief from gases and bloating, there are products like Lactase, lactaid, and other digestive enzymes. So, in this way, one can prevent bloating.

This article contains every discussion on bloating causes and solutions. An overview suggests that excessive production of gastrointestinal gases may cause bloating and abdominal distension. Thus, let's enter the onus of this article. This tells you what food to eat and rules to follow while consuming them in order to prevent bloating after a meal. We would also find that in some people, bloating is psychological. The chronic formation of gases in the digestive system might cause bloating. There are very effective medicines available in today's market which assist in breaking the bubble of gas and wind by collecting them to form a big bubble of gas and getting rid of them by belching or farting.

Post-meal bloating is a common issue that many people go through. It is estimated that bloating symptoms affect a colossal 10 percent of the population. It is a natural process that starts after the meal is consumed. But how much of that is acceptable or appreciable? Thus, we want to percolate it with the causes and the best way to stop bloating after consuming any meal.

1.1. Definition and Symptoms

Overall, bloating remains a commonly described phenomenon with poorly understood pathophysiology. There are numerous intersecting mechanisms that are proposed and studied for bloating including insufficient meal size regulation, slower distal GI transit time, microbial fermentation of food (creating gas), everything possible associated with the local environment in the ileum and colon including stomach volume expansion from swallowed air.

The following are symptoms of bloating, as listed in the Rome IV report: - Sensation of abdominal fullness or pressure - Feeling excessively full after a meal (medically called 'early satiety') - Increased girth of the abdomen (distension) - Abdominal girth fluctuates within the day - Abdominal discomfort: a feeling of swelling or tightness - Decreased overall quality of life due to bloating

Bloating is one of those symptoms that everyone can relate to but may not fully understand. Simply, 'bloating' is the sensation of increased pressure in your abdomen after eating - often accompanied by a visible increase in diameter. This sensation may come from a problem originating within the abdomen or might also be triggered without a real shift in abdominal girth (like the sensation of water retention in pre-menstrual symptoms). The term 'bloating' is used widely and can represent many differing affairs, which is central to why solving the bloating issue is complex. It is advised to be precise when describing bloating as many people will mistake bloating for distension and vice versa. Bloating is a subjective feeling, whilst distension is an objective increase in abdominal girth.

1.2. Prevalence and Impact

Only one study (n = 16) has reported measuring QoL changes during induced acute post-meal bloating. These results showed that bloating added to the negative impact of abdominal pain and the sum of abdominal symptoms, with a significant effect over time for the measurement (Hr impactful). The study by De Maeyer et al. indicates that post-meal bloating makes major contributions to wellbeing and QoL. Eapen et al. demonstrated that post-meal bloating, along with abdominal pain and satisfaction with defecation, predict many components of wellbeing and QoL. Collectively, these data highlight the importance of addressing and preventing high levels of post-meal bloating within the general community. To this end, however, it is crucial to understand the causes of post-meal bloating.

Post-meal bloating, or postprandial bloating, is a common complaint, with research indicating that approximately 18 to 30% of people may develop this symptom within a one-hour postprandial window. Women are consistently shown to be more affected by this phenomenon than men, although results have been mixed with respect to age group. Bloating is the sensation of increased stomach pressure due to retention of gas (flatus and/or swallowed air) and increased fluid/gas in the bowel. Postprandial bloating has significant physical activity-limiting, dietary, and/or social consequences in up to 60% of individuals, with 80% of individuals reporting that it affects their mood. Long-term (24 h), post-meal bloating has consistently been shown to affect quality of life (QoL), usually assessed using the Irritable Bowel Syndrome Quality of Life (IBS-QoL) questionnaire, and overall wellbeing.

2. Digestion Process and Bloating

Bloating can decrease over the course of the day as the body expels some of the gas in the form of belching or the passing of flatus. It can also be a result of swallowing air, which is referred to as aerophagia. Eating too quickly and drinking carbonated drinks are causative situations for swallowing air. Many people report frequent feelings of bloating. Swallowing air and indigestion are common causes of this. Chewing gum, smoking, gastroparesis, and the use of some medications can contribute to bloating, more specifically. Amounts of gas can lead to changes in the composition of the gut flora, fermentation, and abnormal production, which might result in bloating. Scientists and laypersons alike seem to agree that gas in the colon is a frequent source of bloating. Sciatica or a slipped disc is not associated with bloating. Bloating happens in the absence of sharp pain in the lower right part of the stomach. It is not, however, exclusively triggered by increased findings from ultrasound of a filled colon in people with bloating.

Bloating in the stomach is a condition in which the abdomen feels full and tight, while also being swollen. This kind of sensation is usually experienced in the stomach area. Bloating, distension, or the chronic sensation of 'fullness' are excessive occurrences of wind in the colon. A variety of systems in the body can be influenced by excess wind in the colon. Alongside other members of the digestive system (i.e., mouth, esophagus, and stomach), the colon is a part of the digestive process where food is broken down and used as fuel, which means it is a common place for problems such as bloating to occur.

2.1. Overview of Digestive System

The stomach is the first major organ of the GI system and functions as a primary integrator in the processing of food. It is a reservoir for food regulation and also a center for temporal and chemical regulation. In digestion, the stomach acts as a blender in mixing and processing the food. While in the stomach, digestion continues, water, birth, and mix in the form of insoluble particles. Most of the ingested food enters the small intestines two to four hours after ingestion. Once the stomach grinds the food, it empties it as chyme entering the small intestines to be ready for digestion. The time varies depending on the type of meal but typically a normal size meal emptied from the stomach is 6 hours. In distress experience individual, foods take a longer time to empty. The stomach's musculature is responsible for the churning and grinding of the food and moving it ahead to the small intestine for more processing. Retropulsion is the back and forth movement that the food undergoes in the stomach and the valve at the end of the stomach. Only 1 – 2% of the chyme that enters the small intestine is large enough to contain particulates.

The digestive system consists of a long tube called the gastrointestinal (GI) tract. Zooming out to look at the anatomy of the GI system, the mouth where digestion begins, it progresses from the stomach through the small intestine to the colon, and exits through the rectum and anus. The primary function of the GI tract is to break down our food, absorb the nutrients, and excrete what is not absorbable. The process of digestion typically begins in the mouth where mastication occurs. The bolus is then swallowed and passes through the esophagus to the stomach, which secretes chyme. The chyme is released into the small intestines where digestion completes and the nutrients are absorbed into the blood. The non-absorbable substances are then consolidated in the colon and excreted.

2.2. Common Causes of Bloating

As you may now know, bloating can be quite a common occurrence, but it doesn't have to be a totally unavoidable daily burden. By being more conscious of the potential causes listed above, you may be able to reduce the likelihood of bloating happening to you. Eat more slowly. If bloating happens after eating, it may be the result of gulping down meals too quickly. The rapid eating pace tends not to allow time for the body to notify the brain that the stomach is full, causing meal-eaters to overconsume. Drinking through straws is another means of increasing air consumption. Carbohydrates are a major cause of bloating. It's important to know that just because a food item is healthy, that doesn't mean there's no way it could ever cause bloating! Experiment with various "gas-reducing" dietary ideas to see which ones have an impact. Keep an eye out for various foods that could cause gas, whether they are unprocessed or not. In the interim, adding certain foods was discovered to have a casual impact on bloating concerns. Some of these substances include ginger, peppermint, and pineapple. In the not-so-distant future, you may see an increase in the level of digestive comfort.

There are a variety of common causes that can contribute to feelings of bloating after eating. In many cases, bloating is the result of eating too quickly. Consuming food and drinks at a rapid pace can lead to increased air consumption during meals. The presence of extra air in the digestive tract can account for stomach expansion and bloating. Peptic ulcers, cancerous growths, and blockages are other medical concerns that are closely linked to bloating. These health conditions obstruct the movement of food and gas through the digestive system, and as a result, can lead to feelings of fullness and bloating. A dairy allergy or sensitivity can also trigger bloating for some individuals. The discomfort is often related to the body's inability to sufficiently break down lactose into digestive enzymes. The undigested lactose produces a more accommodating environment for bacteria in the intestines, which can make the person feel bloated. Fortunately, dietary changes can help to reduce the likelihood of this happening.

3. Dietary Factors Contributing to Bloating

The main component of swallowed or inhaled air is nitrogen (N2), which makes up about 77% of atmospheric air. Carbon dioxide (CO2) reaches 83 ml/min of resting alveolar ventilation, whereas hydrogen (H2) is practically absent from alveolar air during fasting (3-4 parts per million). As for the causes, post-meal gas is the result of the interaction of multiple endogenous and exogenous factors; the former may act to decrease diatomic nitrogen from the swallowed air to form a single bubble before it reaches the small bowel, favoring its resolution, while the latter act primarily by favoring the production of a greater amount of gas. The main excess gas-producing factors include dietary intake of non-absorbable carbohydrates, dietary fiber, and fructose.

In addition to swallowed or inhaled air, other factors can also contribute to bloating. Of these, dietary factors are a main culprit in the occurrence of post-meal bloating. The following sections shed some light on the main food components and food categories responsible for producing more gas and, in some cases, for slowing gastric emptying. Why does this happen? What symptoms can arise from their consumption in both healthy subjects and in patients with minor and major alterations in functionality? It must be emphasized, however, that most of the studies presented do not specify the quantity of food intake, the duration of the meal, or the maladaptive behaviors in some subjects.

3.1. FODMAPs and Bloating

Foods that are high in FODMAPs include classics such as garlic and onions, but the list also extends to foods like apples and honey. The low-FODMAP diet has been increasingly utilized and studied for the treatment of irritable bowel syndrome. One small study of 40 patients reports that most participants experienced a reduction or resolution of bloating after a 4-week low-FODMAP diet. Socially, eating out or shopping at a grocery store for FODMAP-friendly products can be somewhat challenging due to the necessity of reading labels or preventing knowledge of foods not typically high in Western diets. Researchers are not currently able to predict which individuals are more susceptible to bloating from ingestion of FODMAPs. However, as with any dietary change, symptoms can take hours or days to show up in people, so close observation and planned food reintroductions are necessary to make any conclusions during a trial eating pattern.

Foods that contain FODMAPs (fermentable oligosaccharides, disaccharides, monosaccharides, and polyols) have come under scrutiny in recent years due to their ability to induce bloating and other unpleasant gastrointestinal symptoms. The term FODMAP was coined by researchers at Monash University and serves as an umbrella for describing a collection of molecules or foods that share the common characteristic of being potential gas producers in the digestive system. They are broken down or fermented by bacteria in the colon, and the gas that is released during these bacterial metabolic processes can lead to the feeling of fullness, pain, and bloating. Additionally, for some people, water is also drawn into the gut, which is a way for the body to dilute and remove undigested food products that sit in the small and large intestines.

3.2. High-Fiber Foods

Excess gas after a meal can also be a result of your body not having enough fiber. Fiber helps the body keep moving in a healthy way, which also removes waste. A high-fiber diet that's mainly due to whole foods, including fruits and veggies, supports the formation of stool. Pregnant women with loss of bowel function can benefit from this diet.

On its website, the ACG advises that people try a low-fiber diet if they have no other underlying health concerns except bloating and passing gas, as the first line of defense. This may help to reduce the affliction or lessen its effects. That's because too much fiber is documented as one of the potential "offenders" in a diet that could cause immediate post-meal bloating. "I have my patients reduce their fiber intake because there are some people who simply cannot digest it well," Ioachimescu explains. The recommendation is to put fiber back in after the post-meal distention and gas issues have been resolved—this should be determined by working with a healthcare provider, experts say.

Normally, a high-fiber diet is recommended for a variety of health reasons. Still, there are potential downsides to mostly consuming foods with a high fiber content. Foods like lentils, broccoli, and chickpeas contain a high amount of fiber.

3.3. Carbonated Beverages

There are several factors that can contribute to bloating, and consuming carbonated beverages is one of them. People who frequently feel bloated should carefully observe if carbonated beverages might be the reason. Bloating following a large meal is something that many of us deal with. The source of gas production is the interaction between the carbohydrates, yeast, and bacteria found in these products with the acid already in the stomach. This reaction is responsible for the carbonation in the beverage, the bubbles of which make it difficult for food to be properly digested. When that food is left undigested, it can cause irritation in the upper digestive tract. Solutions for bloating include steering away from beverages other than water, such as acidic compounds, which have been found to decompose very quickly, making it difficult to digest our food. When such beverages are required, consuming a minimum of one glass of water to slow down the decomposition of the acidic beverages is recommended, or including a pinch of baking soda into the beverage for faster acidic compound breakdown.

3.3 Carbonated Beverages

4. Lifestyle Habits and Bloating

Liquid - About 1/3 to 1/2 of your stomach volume is available for food when the stomach is empty so avoid drinking more than 6-8 ounces (200-250ml) of liquid before meals to avoid rapid stomach stretching and pressure on the stomach. Drinking during the meal can also result in a sense of fullness and pressure due to those deep, biological signals that the stomach realizes when it is stretched. To empty "food" liquid from the stomach into the intestine, allow easier passage of gas so ease bloating making belching or flatulence more effective, try to drink most of your liquids 30 minutes before or 30 to 60 minutes after meals. Remember, this is helpful only if there are no rapid emptyers or brisk refluxers. If you have rapid emptying or particularly bad reflux, avoid drinking liquids 30-60 minutes before or after meals.

Eating behaviors - Talking or laughing a lot while eating can also result in air swallowing and contribute to increased gas in your stomach or small intestine. Stress also influences digestion and can lead to motility problems and slower emptying of the stomach.

Ingesting air - Eating or drinking too quickly can result in air swallowing and, therefore, distention. Remove gum-chewing from your list of habits to decrease swallowed air that can contribute to bloating.

Common Causes of Post-Meal Bloating

There are a variety of lifestyle habits that directly impact post-meal bloating, which is the distension or increase in the size of one's abdomen due to gas retention. It is important to address all of the factors that can lead to a bloating episode to be effective in resolving digestive problems. These lifestyle factors include ingesting air, eating behaviors, exercising or drinking large amounts of liquid before, during or after eating, meal sizes, and timing of meals.

4.1. Eating Too Quickly

Mindfulness, called 'dispositional mindfulness', has therefore been studied through a positive psychological lens, leading to new research areas that have benefited from contributions from an array of angles, including business ethics and social engagement. With respect to eating habits, mindful individuals seem to 'be less likely to choose larger portion sizes' and may or may not feel satiated with remarkably smaller quantities of food, when compared to when they eat with other or fewer attention. Given time to reflect upon what we eat allows us to ponder ethical issues related to genetic modification and issues that concern the mass production of what reaches our table. Running in a frenzy to meet a schedule or a meal quickly in order to seize control of a busy next bunch of anticipated chores goes against meditation's antithesis: deliberate motion.

Speeding through a meal is almost a guarantee of bloating. It seems that when we eat fast, we eat more. To appreciate why - and, hopefully, adopt a slower rhythm - let's remind ourselves that a bodily function as critical as selecting, digesting, absorbing and excreting nutrients is too important to be left to the brutality of a hungry stomach seized by a desperate hand putting food in its mouth. Eating foods, beyond their flavor, contributes to our life quality and length, and we would prefer to have control over our food, ensuring that we take in what is needed and in the right proportion. This form of control is a form of mindfulness, an active attention accompanied by observation of our own body. On the other hand, when we actively direct our thoughts to other matters - rather than worrying about food, or at the other end, by feeling overly concerned with it - we may find ourselves overeating.

4.2. Lack of Physical Activity

The next time we consume food, the carbohydrate-to-journey slows until the storage of our glycogen is met, and ultimately slows down. This is the muscle mechanism for reducing the onset of bloating. For those who experience bloating daily, moving on a regular basis is recommended. Walking and swimming are examples of low-impact and/or moderate endurance cardiovascular exercises that use up the glycogen stores out of the liver. As a result, exercising daily can help to decrease gas levels that are tied down in the organs and tissues until the next time of substantial exertion or time of release.

Our muscles store energy, known as glycogen, for use up to 20 minutes after consumption. If the glycogen is not used, it is stored either in the working muscles as a backup, or in the liver, kidney, and nerve cells. Once all these stores are full, any remaining carbohydrates are stored and absorbed as fats. As our organs slow down, glycogen is released as a gas in the form of carbon dioxide and water that is exhaled from the body.

Exercise has many benefits for maintaining digestive health and reducing bloating, specifically. A physically active body has improved glucose regulation, as well as reduced bloating due to improvements to the digestive system. Reduced bloating after meals can be due to a release of gas stored by the muscles and organs in the vicinity of the abdomen. It is this emptying of gases that can help alleviate feelings of post-meal bloating, soreness, cramping, and discomfort. When we are sedentary or inactive, we store gases in the body that might not have been released until hours or days later.

5. Medical Conditions Associated with Bloating

One or more examples of food allergies, intolerance, and allergy overlapping intolerance include lactose intolerance, fructose malabsorption, irritable bowel syndrome (IBS), and gluten-related bloating. Targeted treatment should be carried out to overcome intolerant allergen. Loads of breath-hydrogen tests or the run-out procedure are usually not worthwhile. Patients need to avoid dietary changes guided by the specialists. Interestingly, these patients often suffer elliptocytosis and iron-deficiency anemia before surgery but often improve postpyloric function following anti-reflux surgery performed for cyanosis. Low-caloric food is not universally known. Immunologic tests carried out in some authors have shown that part of the patient suffers post-prandial bloating due to food intolerance. Drug reactions. Some drugs have been linked to post-prandial bloating.

Medical conditions associated with bloating: it is true that numerous factors can produce a feeling of bloatedness. Bloating can occur after eating, but it can also last for long periods of time. Post-prandial bloating is reduced or absent in individuals with gastroparesis. Small bowel distension and slow liquid or solid meal emptying are more common in patients and healthy subjects who report post-prandial bloating. A number of these symptoms are often the result of intestinal and extra-intestinal disorders. Ignoring them can postpone correct diagnosis and the beginning of the appropriate treatment. Although these causes are described as independent of celiac disease, delayed resolution of bloating has been associated with wheat consumption. Any suspected bloating reactions may be the cause of food allergies.

5.1. Irritable Bowel Syndrome (IBS)

Because bloating can frequently accompany different irritability of the gastrointestinal tract, a diet tailored to this purpose might help reduce it (GI). While sensitivity to these foods can vary from person to person, foods associated with IBS symptoms and—importantly—the foods that are associated with the bloating of IBS sufferers on a regular food and bloating diary collected by Castro et al. Several foods have been linked to gas generation, including sugars and carbohydrates in potatoes, apples and stone, severely beaten grains, and processed products such as wheat, legumes such as beans, and, at times, onion. Some indigestible fibers may be a major contributor to bloating, according to recent research, for the World Journal of Gastroenterology. When a person believes that he or she may have bloating connected with irritable bowel syndrome and is diagnosed, a little diet experimentation can help tailor dietary recommendations for that individual person.

Irritable bowel syndrome (IBS), once an unknown condition, has been referred to as a 'diagnostic dilemma', and a 'vexing syndrome'. It is difficult to diagnose because there is no additional available diagnostic examination. Though at some point or another, it is easy to have symptoms or disagreeable results (anyone experience bloating after a vacation feast?). This may create gastrointestinal signs that appear, but the bloating is kept and one simply notices that one is bloated. Query: when do you realize that something is bloating-regularly, after eating or drinking anything in particular? Bloating could be a sign of IBS if it arrives with abdominal discomfort.

In the Nutrients study, 51% of diagnosed celiac disease subjects claimed bloating as a symptom. While bloating is the most common, other digestive symptoms are also present. Gas is a symptom in 45% of diagnosed celiac disease patients. Bloating occurs more often in women than men. Bloating is common in asymptomatic celiac disease patients. While bloating is a common symptom in celiac disease, the root cause is less clear. In observational research appearing in the May 2016 issue of the Colombian Medical Review, researchers highlighted a few ways celiac disease may lead to bloating. Bloating is the result of an overgrowth of bacteria in the small intestine, which is called Small Intestinal Bacterial Overgrowth (SIBO). Celiac disease is a recognized cause of SIBO. Consequently, the Colombian authors suggest stool testing and prescribed antibiotic treatment when necessary. They also recommend that celiac disease patients should go vegetarian (lacto-ovo) because of the lactose intolerance that goes hand in hand with persistent villous atrophy. Host-initiated permanent adherence to a strict gluten-free diet prevents the recurrence of at least most of these problems. This reduces the likelihood of developing an irritable bowel. Therefore choosing a vegetarian lifestyle is unnecessary.

Celiac disease is a hereditary disorder that often interferes with the proper function of the digestive system. Not surprisingly, the symptoms of celiac disease often involve problems of the digestive system. Some classic celiac disease symptoms that involve the digestive system are diarrhea, gas, and bloating. In research published in the September 2018 issue of Nutrients, seven specific digestive symptoms were found to be common among celiac disease patients, with bloating being the most common. The symptoms associated with celiac disease among patients diagnosed late in life were very similar to those that occur in children. Until very recently, it was thought that celiac disease was a disease only of children. A new study showed that at least half of celiac disease patients are currently diagnosed over the age of 45.

6. Prevention and Management Strategies

Chew all your food well to mechanically break it down even further before swallowing. Avoid meals and snacks high in added sugar, artificial sweeteners, and sugar alcohols like those found in low-calorie or reduced-sugar products. Avoid excessive consumption of alcoholic drinks. Increase hydration, at least in part because of low water intake. Compensate for dehydration's role in bloating by focusing on sipping soup, broth, herbal teas, expressing non-caffeine-hot-and-cold combo beverages, such as peppermint or ginger, or hydrating foods, essentially diluting the disproportion of water to sodium that can set you up for that full feeling. And gently move each day – again ideally following by a half-hour or more from each meal or snack – for topical potential to get things "flowing" within your digestive tract. Opt to choose savvy snacks if you're aiming for pain-free digestion, avoiding excessive fat, added sugars, and calories.

Prevention and management strategies. The most effective strategy for managing post-meal bloating is to prevent it in the first place. To do that, begin with these modifications to your dietary habits. Try eating with intention and paying attention to portion sizes. Strive to opt for a high-fiber regime, easing into these changes gradually to give your digestive system and gut microbiome time to adjust. Probiotics can also introduce new healthy bacteria to your gut, focusing on bloating relief with Lactobacillus acidophilus or Bifidobacterium lactis. Regardless, reach out to your healthcare provider for their recommendations before starting a new supplement. You may also explore digestive enzymes, either through eating vegetables raw or in their gut-friendly, "tamed" forms — anything from cucumber to your favorite root vegetables.

6.1. Dietary Modifications

As a dietician or an informed consumer, the following general dietary strategies may be helpful in managing post-meal bloating: - Breaking up with sugar alcohols and high fructose corn syrup (HFCS) - Decreasing portion sizes: larger portion sizes, particularly of high-fat and high-fiber foods, result in more bloating - Minimizing carbonation - Eliminating chewing gum - Altering protein portion: aim for protein-rich foods at each meal with the inclusion of small to moderate servings of the protein-based item (e.g. grilled chicken, tempeh, edamame, cheese) rather than large servings of beans, chili, lentils, or seitan - Managing cruciferous and allium-rich vegetables - Managing phytates-containing grains and legumes - Managing dairy with food products that contain lactose - Eating smaller portions of food in a more relaxed manner rather than bolus eating - Several commonly used dietary habits and foodstuffs may be making postprandial bloating worse. Proactively supporting patients to make the above-mentioned dietary changes may reduce the likelihood of bloating.

Given that gas production is often a strong contributor to bloating, addressing dietary behaviors is an area primed for intervention. It's difficult to create comprehensive guidelines for dietary modifications that can decrease bloating because there is ample individual variability in food tolerance. However, several modifications can be made to reduce the amount of gas produced by colonic fermentation. Enzymatic breakdown of fermentable substrates by gut bacteria yields gas within the gut lumen. Limiting intake of those substrates means that less gas will be released as a result of these fermentation processes. Reduction of carbohydrate is particularly effective in managing IBS or IBS symptoms.

6.2. Probiotics and Digestive Enzymes

These enzymes are sold as "systemic" formulas, which can help ease bloating, gastrointestinal symptoms, and exhaustion that some customers may feel after a significant meal. In reality, according to a 2011 study in the World Journal of Gastroenterology, healthy individuals taking the enzyme alpha-galactosidase, which breaks down complex carbohydrates found in fiber, beans, and greens, reported a decrease in bloating. For a non-over-the-counter solution, a healthcare professional may conduct a blood or breath test to verify food sensitivities such as lactose or fructose. These assessments measure how long the stomach requires to digest certain meals. Food sensitivities, which may cause or worsen bloating, can draw the above solutions.

Though not all supplements have concrete evidence of their efficacy for post-meal bloating, it is possible that some might aid in managing it. After eating, beneficial bacteria and other microorganisms living in the gut process food particles that the body has trouble digesting. Over the counter, probiotics might transplant a variety of helpful bacteria species into the intestines. Available evidence shows that they can alleviate symptoms of post-meal bloating as well as other abdominal discomforts. Digestive enzymes, which help the body break down big food particles into smaller, more comfortable tasks, are widely available in chain drugstores.

7. Seeking Professional Help

These tests are used to assess how quickly food moves through the stomach and into the upper portion of the intestines. In those experiencing a delay in stomach emptying, the amount of pressure in the intestines and the rate at which those muscles contract are often below the average. Additionally, the test can be used to examine how well the stomach may assimilate certain nutrients.

Gastroenterologists often diagnose and manage bloating. However, if doctors suspect disorders or conditions outside the gastrointestinal (GI) tract, they may consult with and refer individuals to other specialists such as cardiologists or endocrinologists. Begin a conversation with a healthcare professional when bloating is a recurring symptom, causes worry or inconveniences, leads to impairment in an individual's social life, family life, interpersonal relationships, or ability to work, causes moderate to severe anxiety, or is accompanied by unintentional weight loss. In cases of severe diarrhea or blood in stool, a visit to the emergency department may be necessary. The following tests may be recommended by doctors.

In some cases, bloating can interfere with daily life or suggest an underlying issue. Those struggling with the feeling of being bloated more often than not may also want to consult with a healthcare professional about treatments and self-care practices suited to their individual needs. Considering the following symptoms, factors, and causes may help doctors arrive at an appropriate diagnosis and treatment plan. While bloating can have a wide range of causes, functional GI disorders - in particular - are commonly associated with the symptom. If they suspect such a condition, doctors may recommend the following to diagnose bloating:

7.1. When to Consult a Healthcare Provider

When a person chews on simethicone pills, they turn the mini bubbles of natural gas into greater ones, which are then more readily forfeited within a flush from the bowels. To alleviate the pain, people may take OTC medications.

In the early stages, bloating, stomach ache, as well as gas may be cured by utilizing a heating pad, wandering in gentle motion, and performing some workouts. Over-the-counter remedies for ache and puff might also be tried whenever house therapies don't manage bloating. Examples of these goods incorporate: - Pepto-Bismol, which holds the active substance bismuth subsalicylate - Simethicone pills include Gas-X, Mylanta Gas Relief, as well as others

Suitable treatments for gas

Bloating often resolves on its own, with the aid of over-the-counter treatments for gas and pain; however, people can consult with a healthcare provider if they still have bloating even after a month or longer. Call a healthcare provider right away if the bloating takes place together with the following: - Lack of hunger - Unexplained weight loss (loss of 5% of body weight within a six-month time frame) - Dark, tarry stools - Chronic diarrhea - Serious or debilitating abdominal discomfort - Bloating that lasts a month or longer - Nausea or vomiting - Shortness of breath or difficulty breathing - Weariness, lethargy, or jaundice

Summary

People should also seek medical advice if bloating does not resolve after two or three days of rest, at-home treatments, or OTC medications.

Call a doctor if bloating occurs alongside any of the following signs or symptoms: - Loss of appetite - Unexplained weight loss - Black, tarry stools - Persistent diarrhea - Persistent bloating - Nausea or vomiting - Shortness of breath or difficulty breathing - Unexplained fatigue or weakness - Swelling in the abdomen, legs, or other areas of the body - Persistent, severe, or worsening abdominal pain

Most of the time, bloating resolves on its own, or it may also be reduced from at-home treatments, such as applying a heating pad to the stomach or drinking water. Some healthcare professionals recommend seeking medical evaluation if a person is experiencing any bloating-related pain or continues to experience bloating every day for one month. People should also discuss their symptoms with a healthcare professional whenever there are red-flag indicators of a serious underlying condition.

Reducing bloating

7.2. Diagnostic Tests for Bloating

In some individuals, cathartic and emetic (vomiting) doses of narcotic d-phenylalanine and/or a d/l amino add mixture may be prescribed as a test to ultimately indicate whether a guide to the stomach by removing the drug that is bulk-related. Radiographic tests to determine not only transit, but also stomach volumes in fasting and full states follow rather than simply evaluate transit: antroduodenal manometry, gastric emptying scintigraphy, and gastric emptying breath tests, performed with a radiotelemetric capsule (smartpill). In these cases, the bowel is being used as a passive transmitter of a dose administered in one location, the stomach. Such tests can show normal transit but an impaired accommodation response, which can only be evaluated with meal challenges in manometry or intraluminal pressure recording (with gastric and small amplitude or sometimes also length) sensors. More recent tests using endoplus are also now being performed.

In patients who experience bloating, a healthcare provider typically performs a complete physical examination. This allows for the necessary tests that can lead to a diagnosis. To further identify post-meal bloating, which may take place for any number of reasons such as dietary triggers, bacterial overgrowth or disordered transit, hydrogen breath tests for fructose, lactose, sucrose, lactulose, whole body glucose, and/or d-xylose may be administered by physicians. A problem with the hydrogen breath tests is that they may yield false-positive or false-negative results and can produce positive results in healthy individuals who do not have symptoms, because the test looks for bacterial metabolism of saccharides with their release of hydrogen or methane. In a healthy group, these tests may have 6-50% false-positive results. Given that results can be difficult to interpret, any ultimate treatment plan should also be based on response of the patient to specific therapy.

8. Conclusion and Key Takeaways

- Bloating solutions: - Testing for intolerance and addressing an underactive stomach or indigestion - Limiting high-fermentation foods to a moderate amount every few days - Consuming smaller meals - Addressing candida and ensuring adequate bile flow

- Frequent causes of bloating: - Carbohydrate malabsorption or bacterial overgrowth in the intestine - Food intolerance including fructose and lactose intolerance - Secondary effect of mitochondrial dysfunction, food sensitivities, or inflammation - Inefficient digestion due to inadequate stomach acid or inconsistent food combinations - Nervous indigestion resulting in delayed bowel transit

Bloating after a meal can be confusing and frustrating because it is challenging to pinpoint the cause and subsequently fix it. However, today we have been able to shed more light on the issue by discussing the various possible causes and their corresponding solutions. Furthermore, we have analyzed bloating from various angles including bacterial overgrowth, intolerance to specific carbohydrates, starches, and fibers in fruits and vegetables, secondary effects brought about by mitochondrial dysfunction and/or food sensitivities, and poor transitioning of the food from the stomach to the gut or inadequate mixing between food and digestive juices. Finally, we have discussed complementary remedies to alleviate any bloating not caused by an underlying problem. These factors should help you explore what might be causing your bloating and help you better understand how you can alleviate it. We have covered a lot of ground, so to summarize, here is everything in bullet point form:

Understanding and Managing Stomach Bloating After Eating

1. Introduction to Stomach Bloating

Stomach bloating is a common concern for many people. Many people have reported stomach bloating in their lives, which makes the condition a common one. Bloating can occur for a variety of causes, including trapped gas, consumption of certain foods, general digestive issues, or a chronic condition known as irritable bowel syndrome. Though bloating is usually harmless, research suggests that retaining fluid in the stomach may impair one's way of life, create mental stress, or even lead to serious discomfort in some cases. A doctor can help a person connect a bloating episode to a particular cause while ruling out more ambiguous symptoms of other digestive issues. Managing bloating as it occurs or preventing it in the first place are both important strategies. However, if bloating causes discomfort, visit a healthcare provider to ensure that it doesn't interfere with a person's eating habits.

Stomach bloating: You know the feeling. It can be uncomfortable and lead to discomfort and distress. In the following sections, we'll go over the causes of bloating, how it impacts the body, when to see a doctor, and how to handle it. It's not unusual for bloating to follow a meal. There are different variables that can induce bloating after eating. Learn what they are and how to manage them in this blog. This piece examines the physical health issue of stomach bloating, which is sometimes used interchangeably with "abdominal distention" to refer to trapped gas or air in the stomach or intestines. The appearance or feeling of fullness can accompany it. Some people mistake bloating for water weight, but they are distinct phenomena.

1.1. Definition and Causes of Stomach Bloating

Stomach bloating occurs as a result of three primary causes: swallowed air, natural gas, and food remnants that have not yet been digested. The immediate remedy for stomach bloating is the management of the cause. When stomach bloating results from swallowed air, the best thing an individual can do is release the air by either belching or flatulating. If the air is causing occasional discomfort, breathing in half an hour is a cure. When bloating is brought on by a gas-producing food habit, the individual partaking of the meal should abstain from such food. If constipation is the problem, the person should boost their fiber and fluid intake and engage in physical activity to encourage abdominal movement. Meals should be taken at regular intervals to avoid missing out on the process of defecation. In addition, doctors may prescribe system relaxation approaches and adjustments to the individual's bowel activity.

Stomach bloating is a condition that is characterized by the uncomfortable sensation of abdominal distension after eating. This article explores the meaning of stomach bloating and its specific causes. Stomach bloating is when a person feels a full and tight abdomen that may become uncomfortable or painful. It frequently occurs after eating, and flatulence and belching generally accompany it. While it may resemble a buildup of gas in the stomach, bloating most commonly occurs in the abdomen. It is vital for a person to recognize just what they mean when they use the expression "bloating." Flatulence, or passing gas out of the anus, refers to the act of passing gas out of the body.

2. Common Causes of Stomach Bloating After Eating

Note what you ate, how the food was prepared or cooked, condiments, snacks, and any drinks consumed, as well as the time of eating and onset of bloating. This can help you identify which food is to blame for your bloating. Then, avoid that food or limit its intake, and see if your bloating goes away. Consult a doctor. No one deserves to suffer, and unfortunately, your symptoms can sometimes point to bigger issues such as irritable bowel syndrome, celiac disease, or a small intestinal bacterial overgrowth (SIBO). Making lifestyle changes such as stress reduction, consuming live active cultures (or probiotics), and eating fresh, whole foods instead of processed, packaged, convenience foods can also be effective.

Common causes of stomach bloating after eating: - Swallowing air when eating - Consuming carbonated beverages - Eating rapidly - Chewing gum - Lactose intolerance (inability to digest milk sugar) - Fructose intolerance (inability to digest fruit sugar) - Over-the-counter fiber supplements (such as Metamucil) - Drinking through a straw - Malabsorption of sugars, which can be caused by certain medical conditions and diseases

If you frequently experience bloating after eating, it can have a significant impact on your quality of life. Thankfully, establishing a pattern of when bloating occurs, as well as keeping a food diary to track foods consumed, can help identify the trigger of this distressing and uncomfortable symptom.

2.1. Overeating

Because postprandial bloating is poorly studied, the published data are mostly on bloating in general rather than specifically related to meals. In one study of 500 adults in the U.K., 65% of men and 76% of women reported bloating (overall more common in younger adults but not correlated with body mass index) but did not say if their bloating was food-related. The same study found 11% of adults complained of food intolerance, most commonly dairy, spices, citrus, onions, fatty foods, bread, and sugar, which is more focused on the abdomen than general bloating.

Overeating is one of the leading causes of stomach bloating after eating. When we consume too much food in one meal, our digestive tract can become overloaded, leading to excessive fermentation, which in severe cases is clinically diagnosed as a gut bacterial overgrowth or methane-producing constipation. When the gut stretches, the blood supply to the gut decreases and the muscles of the GI system are obstructed, resulting in digestive discomfort and bloating. The intake of excessive calories is quickly converted to energy or avoided as fat but can overwhelm the digestive system that has more limited capacity and deprive the gut tissues of needed blood supply to process the nutrients. The medical term for bloating that is attributed to food or food portions is called postprandial bloating.

2.2. Eating Too Quickly

In other words, inhaling extra air during meals can lead to bloating. Another consequence of eating too quickly is swallowing bits of food that haven't been thoroughly chewed. These partial food particles may not be readily broken down in the stomach. Instead, they may enter the small intestine, where they can ferment quickly. This rise in bacterial activity can produce hydrogen gas, leading to bloating. Reducing the amount of air you swallow at meals, and chewing your food slowly to further reduce swallowed air, may aid in preventing post-meal bloating. The process of swallowing has two distinct aspects, one which we can control and another which is instinctual. For example, during medical procedures or when people are dehydrated, you can suppress swallowing even if you have saliva in your mouth. Therefore, it is relatively easy to suppress eating or drinking when you remember that you are supposed to be avoiding doing so. On the other hand, once you start to chew or drink, the swallowing mechanism becomes more reflexive.

When you eat too quickly, it is natural to inhale a lot of air. You could swallow a lot of this if you are simultaneously sipping a carbonated beverage. While some gas will exit your body in the form of a burp, other gas will travel through your digestive system, carrying partially digested food particles with it. This is bound to make your stomach feel expanded.

2.3. Food Intolerances and Sensitivities

Histamine, including in foods, can lead to symptoms of bloating. In addition to an actual food intolerance, some foods may contain biogenic amines, including histamine. These naturally-occurring compounds accumulate in inappropriately stored foods. Some common biogenic amine-containing foods include alcohol, avocado, some cheeses, cured meats, and smoked meats/fish. One of the more frequently asked questions is, "What can I eat?" I recommend keeping a detailed food diary for ten to fourteen days and then also monitor for times of bloating. Being able to see your food in black and white sometimes helps identify potential patterns in your life.

Food Sensitivities

High consumption of sugar alcohol, which is used as a non-nutritive sweetening agent, can lead to symptoms of stomach bloating after its ingestion. People frequently experience adverse effects after consuming sugar alcohols, including xylitol, sorbitol, and mannitol. Additionally, lactose intolerant individuals may experience similar symptoms due to intolerance of lactose added to some salad dressings or to dairy used as an ingredient in various food choices. Some food choices contain non-nutritive sweetening agents in their foods, including gum and mints. High volume or large amounts of foods or liquids can lead to bloating. Additionally, the use of carbonated beverages, liquids with caffeine, and alcohol or caffeine that helps with bowel movements can lead to bloating as well. Some wheat, some breweries in beer processors, can lead to gastrointestinal symptoms and bloating without gluten.

Food Intolerances

3. Gut Health and Stomach Bloating

Overall, it contributes to a healthier immune system and the growth of stomach cells. Conversely, stomach problems could arise from an unhealthy gut. After eating any form of food, the food that is undigested reaches the large intestine of the human stomach because of various reasons, in which the microflora present in the gut acts on it to digest it. However, the undigested part consists of many natural gases which are liberated at the end by the action of gut microflora. In people with an unhealthy and irregular gut system, this gas can lead to stomach bloating. Bacteria in the gut produce carbon dioxide, hydrogen, and methane when they feed on gas as a byproduct while consuming food as a substrate (bacterial energy source). In order to maintain a high level of gastrointestinal function, the number of gut microbiota is kept low. Probiotics are also some of the gut microbiota which contribute to a healthy stomach.

Gut health and stomach bloating are intricately connected. The balance and types of gut microbiotas present in the gastrointestinal (GI) tract play a crucial role in digestion. When food reaches the stomach, the enzymes break it down into simpler compounds such as carbohydrates and proteins, which are then further degraded in the small intestine. Species such as Actinobacteria, Firmicutes, and other microorganisms present in the gut maintain the equilibrium in the gut and are needed to maintain its proper functioning. If everything is in order, it will help one to absorb essential nutrients from the food. Gut health is very important to maintain an overall healthy body as a high number of microbiota synthesize a number of beneficial compounds which include vitamin K and some of the vitamin B forms.

3.1. Role of Gut Microbiota in Digestion

The balance between different microorganisms in the gut is what will influence the digestion of food. If the gut has more good or beneficial microorganisms, then digestion will be faster and more complete. The good bacteria will also consume particles that are left behind, helping to minimize fermentation. In this case, the symptoms of bloating may be lower. However, if the balance of good and bad bacteria is altered, digestion will be incomplete, leading to slower digestion in the colon, which is what will promote fermentation, as bad bacteria will grow and have food to consume. Gas released from the bacteria will make the walls of the colon expand and contract faster, which is what will then cause bloating. The larger the quantity of undigested food that enters into the colon, the more gas will be produced, and therefore the worse the symptoms of bloating can become. Similarly, if the individual consumes a high carbohydrate diet, digestion delays carbohydrate digestion and will cause fermentation, leading to more bloating. If nutrients are absorbed in the small intestine, then good and bad bacteria will have almost no chance to grow.

When food in the stomach has been partially digested, it is released into the small intestine. In the small intestine, enzymes slowly continue to break down the partly digested food to prepare it for absorption as nutrients. Once the food has become small enough, the small intestine will start to absorb and assimilate these basic units. Finally, digested food is moved from the small intestine to the colon, which is the body's main digestive system.

4. Dietary Strategies to Reduce Stomach Bloating

Here's how some dietary changes can help reduce bloating: Reduce fiber content, as higher fiber intakes in some individuals can increase gas production. For example, resistant starch which is found in an excessive quantity in cooked and cooled foods and beans as a high fiber food item. Consuming mostly proteins and fats which are low in fermentable carbs and rarely increase bloating. Making the diet more plant-based. Including plants does not mean that someone has to eat more raw vegetables because not all vegetables are the same in their impact. For instance, excessive gas production is associated with some varieties of lettuce whereas spinach is not known to cause bloating at all. In addition to plant variety, personal tolerances vary. Consuming sufficient omega-3 fatty acids found in seeds, nuts, fish and avocados or taking omega supplement. Reducing artificial sweeteners. Reducing milk products will give an idea of the effectiveness of this particular sugar reduction. These steps will help determine which fermentable carbs may increase someone's bloating. Advisably, focusing on drinking water for hydration instead of tea, coffee, sports drinks and flavored water without artificial sweeteners during these tests.

Including adequate dietary strategies in daily life may reduce the symptoms in the long term. In this section, we outline general dietary changes that may be helpful in reducing stomach bloating. These include consuming less gassy foods, smaller meals and snacks, well-cooked (instead of raw) vegetables and some grains, and staying well hydrated. Reducing bloating involves the conscious and consistent selection of specific foods with two main dietary strategies. The first strategy is to avoid high fiber content, while the second is to prioritize or avoid certain fermentable carbohydrates.

4.1. Fiber Intake and Digestive Health

Suppose you are already consuming about 35 grams and you still have digestive complaints such as digestive pain and bloating after eating. In that case, look at the size of the food that can accumulate and ferment. Try smaller and more frequent meals. You should also use the fatigue system, which relaxes and loosens the muscles in the digestive system. After breakfast, make sure that 10 minutes is enough to run, walk, or practice yoga. These are additional strategies to consider if you continue to experience bloating and stomach pain after eating. Fiber is an important part of a healthy diet, but for those who do not adhere to fiber recommendations, take special care to reduce bloating and other side effects. Many individuals experience bloating, indigestion, and abdominal pain after eating. However, steps can be taken to mitigate these risks.

We go for months without any stomach bloating symptoms. However, when they do hear from people with bloating problem, they say that dietary fiber is hardly mentioned as a solution for overcoming this common complaint. Despite the importance of fiber in good digestive comfort, they continually experience many complaints caused by insufficient intake. There are some people who do not finish the planning process on time not being blamed for not wanting to eat vegetables and fruits? Many who plan their meals tend to enjoy the choice of wheat bread and cereals when fooling around. I believe reasons like these make it difficult. Not only is this nutritional direction of between 23 and 38 grams of fiber they need to sacrifice the minimum recommended and not likely.

4.2. FODMAP Diet

In addition, non-LFDs also had exclusion criteria of poorly absorbed carbohydrates but failed to reduce gastrointestinal symptoms, suggesting that avoidance of high quality evidence suggests an optimal dietary treatment may involve more than lowering delivery of poorly absorbed sugars. More RCTs have been published that have evaluated pediatric or adult effects of an LFD. Following five case-control or cross-sectional studies previously included, our review analyzes an additional three studies, with two of these exploring the effects of LFD in cohort populations. A number of these studies specifically explored bloating as a primary outcome, with a trend towards improvement seen in 9 out of 15 studies, while 9 also observed improvements in other gastrointestinal outcomes. However, many RCTs have methodological weaknesses and contain small sample sizes making inferences difficult.

A low-FODMAP (Fermentable Oligosaccharides, Disaccharides, Monosaccharides, and Polyols) diet (LFD) is an evidence-based dietary approach for the management of functional gut symptoms, such as pain, bloating, diarrhea, fecal urgency, and flatulence. Its theory is based on the idea that reducing the intake of these fermentable carbohydrates in predisposed individuals with irritable bowel syndrome (IBS) can reduce their symptoms by limiting the osmotic laxative effect and discomfort from gas production. Two recent studies have shown that a dietitian-delivered LFD can improve bloating in people with IBS. This suggests that dietary restriction of FODMAPs might reduce bloating independent of diagnosed gastrointestinal disorders.

5. Lifestyle Changes for Managing Stomach Bloating

Regular exercising increases diaphragmatic activity, gives the impression of balancing the resistance of the blood in the abdomen, facilitating the emptying of the stomach and stopping the sensation of bloating. It is recommended that bloating or cramping should be avoided during your workout. Instead, walking or any other mild exercise is recommended. We are special entities, and our response is distinct, and these lifestyle modifications may require a persistent examination of how they can help me. Studies suggest that dietary choices, such as consuming a more plant-centric eating pattern with moderately higher salt quality, bold-flavored meals could minimize bloating. Also, all of these meals are less bloated with white bread and fried food, as well as higher in soluble fiber, fat and protein. A registered dietitian can help you develop an eating plan that works for your personal wellness objectives and tastes.

If you want to decrease your abdominal bloating, you might want to make an effort to incorporate a few changes to your lifestyle. Eating so-called "mindful eating" or "eating with intention" can greatly reduce bloating. This practice restricts frivolous eating and instead concentrates on the food we eat. Slow chewing and eating after a food craving, ideally in a relaxed atmosphere, and feeling pleasant can help improve digestion and prevent bloating.

5.1. Eating Mindfully

Mindful eating maintains a relaxed awareness. We focus on the immediate experience of eating, we do not judge ourselves about what we are eating and do not daydream, conceptualize, or analyze. As we incorporate eating mindfully into our lives, we notice that our digestive system feels better, in general, and we notice a reduction in bloating after the meal or other negative stomach and digestive symptoms. Mindful eating does not ignore the larger picture of changing what you eat, knowing the portion that your body responds best to, or if you need help from a health professional. It is the root to allowing the body and mind to realize, measure, and incorporate changes.

Mindful eating is a concept that advocates using all the senses while eating, being attentive to listening to the body's hunger and satiety cues, and letting go of negative emotions around food. While no research has directly evaluated and/or studied the role of mindful eating practices in reducing bloating, given that these strategies can lead to a relaxation response in the body, it could be considered that mindful eating has positive effects on your digestive well-being. Our gut is known as our second brain as it is filled with nerves that are always signaling to your brain. How your gut feels might be dependent on how you are responding to these signals and to feelings and thoughts.

3.3. Nutritional Support with Probiotic Use There are some problems experienced when probiotics started to be administered. Many gas problems occur particularly in the early periods of use. Patients are often hesitant to use probiotics because they cause excessive gas due to toxicity. There are now many probiotics groups in the market. It should be noted that not every probiotic may be suitable for the person's benefit. It is possible to search and find the most suitable option from commercially available brands. It is appropriate to use lactic acid bacteria and bifidobacterium-enriched products. As a general principle, it would be beneficial to use probiotics with a high content of cetraxanax. Probiotic use allows the reduction of complaints up to 50-70% at most. Although it does not have a full effect, more substantial results will be obtained. In a fresh intestine, there is not only tuning. We can think of the abdomen as a chamber. Like all chambers, there is constantly a flow of the stomach. If a person with regular bowel habits stays at a maximum of 4-5 chambers during prolonged fasting periods and then at the toilet, the expiration phase does not remove the gas and complaints of swelling and rumbling are experienced. When a person stays hungry for a long time and eats afterwards, time should be mobilized to start bowel movements for the process it has started. This will prevent swelling and rumbling complaints. Belly swelling and bloating expand; physical exercises are necessary. Movements affect your stomach and stomach's exit rate. The effect of exercises increases in association with nutrition. For this reason, physical exercises in the absence of regulation on nutrition will not be efficient to alleviate the application. A system with a day-to-day organization is constructed with products with a Special Formula for Individual Needs.

Regular physical activity is vital for managing the health of the digestive system, which is fundamental in controlling bloating. Our digestive system is regulated by the nervous system. Any activity that calms the brain has a positive effect on the digestive system. Headaches, palpitations, anorexia, and body swelling often occur in the case of digestive system problems. It contributes to our overall digestive comfort. Aerobic-type exercise routines that can be performed almost every day of the week have benefits for reducing gut discomfort. Cardiorespiratory exercises tend to stimulate the elimination of gases from the body. The muscles supporting the abdominal organs also work with these exercises. This facilitates the elimination of gas. It is recommended that physical activity be done to reduce the complaints. For example, it would be very useful to apply walking practice immediately after meals. A 30-minute regular walk per day will help reduce complaints.

6. Medical Conditions Associated with Stomach Bloating

Additionally, there are four areas that may be affected in the human body as a result of bloating, including chest, abdomen, pelvis, and generalized whole body (or constitutional).

In addition, chronic idiopathic constipation as a consequence of slow parts of the intestines does not help those who suffer from bloating because they are likely to pass wind more slowly. Aside from the bowels, the digestive system as a whole can also be affected. Particularly, bloating and wind can be experienced quite frequently by people who have adjusted to symptoms of eating gluten before. Gluten is a protein that is found in grains such as wheat, barley, and rye. Coeliac disease is the name of a health condition in which the small intestine is hypersensitive to gluten. Whenever someone with coeliac disease eats gluten, the inside lining of their gut becomes inflamed, leading to malabsorption of nutrients. In turn, digestive symptoms can occur, which renders bloating.

Conditions cause bloating: Medical conditions associated with bloating may be categorized into three places, including the bowels, digestion, and metabolism. Starting with the bowels: it is estimated that irritable bowel syndrome (IBS) is a very common digestive condition which is a long-term problem but cannot be cured fully. Symptoms of IBS can change from person to person. For instance, one person might have severe bloating and abdominal pain but have constipation, whereas another person might suffer from excessive wind alongside diarrhea.

There is quite a lot of information on the topic of bloating. From which foods to eat to avoid it, to links with medical conditions, there is much to discuss.

6.1. Irritable Bowel Syndrome (IBS)

Symptoms depend on the individual and may change frequently. As well as cramping and bloating, people with IBS may also experience a change in bowel habits (diarrhea, constipation, an alternation between the two), gassiness, and sometimes urgent bowel movements. Bloating may be caused by changes in the way the abdominal muscles contract, increased or decreased levels of certain chemicals in the brain and nervous system, or the flow of food or gases within the intestines. Bloating has also been linked to the unhealthy balance of microorganisms within the gut. Therefore, bloating may result from a broad array of digestive system changes, both those of special relevance to people with IBS and those related to the basic digestive functions. The possibility of a diagnosis is important because poorly managing the irritable bowel can lead to a lifetime of bloating and other symptoms.

IBS is also known as "spastic colon" or "spastic colitis." It is a recurrent, incurable, and lifelong condition, requiring long-term treatment and lifestyle management. The irritable bowel is the most common disorder diagnosed by gastroenterologists and one of the most common disorders seen by primary care physicians. Because of its widespread acceptance as a "less serious" disorder, people are often embarrassed or reluctant to report their symptoms. This leads to undue suffering for many.

- Gas in the stomach that is making you feel full and gaseous (this is often caused by swallowing air) - Food reactions (e.g., lactose intolerance, food allergies, celiac disease) - Irritable bowel syndrome (IBS) - Motility problems (e.g., gastroparesis, partial bowel obstruction) - Inflammatory bowel disease

Stomach bloating is an extremely common symptom, and the vast majority of people who experience bloating do not have serious underlying illness. Each person's individual pattern will help determine the actual diagnosis and treatment plan. Common causes of bloating are:

6.2. Celiac Disease

Worldwide, there are varying estimates. Studies point to up to 1 in 100 people may have celiac per general population. The numbers might be even higher if one counts only symptoms of the bowel. The good news is that celiac disease can be treated. The evidence criteria to classify celiac have been substantially revised and should lead to the diagnosis being significantly broadened if incorporated into clinical practice. There are no drugs on the market to help. The excellent news is that if an individual has celiac disease and goes on a strict gluten-free diet, symptoms can get better. Bloating should disappear, although this takes very close attention to any and all foods consumed to make certain that they, too, are gluten-free. Over time, the intestine will heal and the body will start to absorb food. The increased content inside the intestines will decrease and the bloating starts to resolve.

Celiac disease is a condition in which some or all of the protein gluten is toxic to the body. One of the results of consuming gluten in an individual with celiac disease is bloating. When a person with celiac disease consumes food or products containing gluten, the body has an immune response. A section of the small intestine lining produces antibodies which causes inflammation and makes the inner lining flatten out. This, in turn, decreases the surface area, also decreasing the body's capacity to absorb nutrients. A bloated tummy is not the only symptom that may occur when consuming gluten. A person may also have considerable abdominal pain, constipation and/or diarrhea, among other symptoms. These symptoms are not only bothersome but also can lead to a number of other concerning health conditions that research has shown can be associated with celiac disease.

7. When to Seek Medical Advice for Stomach Bloating

In summary, it is important that anyone with unrelenting, progressive bloating no longer considers this a 'normal' part of the aging process, that nothing can be done about. Discussing with a healthcare professional will be able to rule out any serious underlying cause and provide an appropriate and effective management strategy at an earlier stage.

- Blood in your stools or dark tarry stools. Bleeding close to the anus can give you a red-blood mixed-in-with your stool 'fresh' bleed, but if you get dark tarry stools, this means the blood has traveled from higher up your digestive tract and is digested, so needs to be treated as a more serious concern. The blood may not necessarily be from the stomach; however, most blood will make you feel unwell and could indicate a more serious concern. Blood in the stools can be associated with certain types of IBS or Inflammatory Bowel Disease; however, it would likely also be accompanied by other symptoms such as a change in the color, consistency, or frequency of stools and abdominal pain. Blood in the stools can also be caused by celiac disease, so it is always worth seeking help from your healthcare professional to rule out serious conditions.

- Unexplained unintentional weight loss. This is a very non-specific symptom, but when associated with bloating, could indicate a more serious problem such as a malignant disease.

- Unpleasant twisting/tugging sensation. Food passing down the stomach should take about half an hour, and passing through the small intestine should take about three hours. If you have had a meal and then get an uncontrollable twisting, tugging sensation over the next few hours, this could be a sign of a small bowel obstruction. The gut starts off being very soft and floppy, but as the meal progresses, it will gradually get harder and pass through the bowel. Any narrowing, the point of obstruction, means that the normal progression of softer to hard food in the bowel will be interrupted, causing the twisting/tugging problem.

- Bloating is associated with a change in bowel habit. Eating stimulates the gastro-colic reflex, which in turn stimulates colon motility. Therefore, a pre-existing pathology that can drive colonic motility would be more likely to trigger bloating when eating.

Severe bloating and abdominal pain can be a cause for serious concern. It is particularly important to seek medical attention if:

7.1. Persistent or Severe Symptoms

- Progressive worsening of symptoms (occurring over several weeks-months-year) – Bloating that progressively worsens over time may be associated with weight loss, decreased appetite, or early satiety. Generally, symptoms that limit activities despite proper management should raise an alarm for further investigation. - Association with other symptoms – Bloating along with other symptoms in the abdomen such as persistent changes in bowel habit, abdominal pain, rectal bleeding, persistent diarrhea or constipation, vomiting are termed 'red flags'. These cases will warrant investigations via endoscopic means or imaging studies. - Past medical history – A person who has had a history of stomach or colon cancer, significant weight loss, long duration of heartburn and bloating, and has a past surgical history on his/her stomach and bowels should forthwith see a doctor for a thorough work-up. - Gender, age or family history – Unintended weight loss, blood in stool, and bloating; especially in women, unexplained anemia, family history of bowel diseases such as bowel cancer may signal the need for further work up. - Severity – Severe bloating in the chest associated with shortness of breath will warrant same-day review and possible history taking and a physical examination by a healthcare professional.

Signs and symptoms of stomach bloating are usually mild, self-limiting, and will resolve without treatment. It is usually a result of the digestion and fermentation of food within our bowel. However, factors must be taken into consideration when symptoms persist longer than expected, worsen over time, or when symptoms could no longer be managed with olpin or occur along with other symptoms. These cases listed below warrant medical attention for a thorough evaluation.

8. Conclusion and Key Takeaways

If you experience bloating specifically after consuming sugary and/or artificially sweetened items (a diet high in FODMAPs), you should consider seeing a gastroenterologist. Your stool may need to be checked, you may need to be tested for carbohydrate malabsorption (such as lactose malabsorption), you may need an abdominal CT scan to check for constipation or pelvic disorders, and you may need anemia testing or endoscopy for a blood test. You can call the doctor if you're still having digestive problems, you have unexplained weight loss, or you're experiencing discomfort or diarrhea. We've covered a lot. Here are your key takeaways outlined: Understanding Stomach Bloating: An Introduction Common Causes of Stomach Bloating 10 Uncommon and Rare Causes of Stomach Bloating Abdominal Distension vs. Bloating How to Treat Stomach Bloating NSTextAlignment Strategies Balloon Strategies Grocery Shopping Strategies Food and FODMAP Strategies Supplement and Diet Strategies

In summary, you've learned that stomach bloating often occurs as a result of swallowed air, bacterial fermentation in the gut, IBS, or food intolerance. It is a result of gas or fluid entering the digestive tract and has many causes, including poor dietary habits. It can be related to abdominal distension and can be managed by altering your diet, behavior, thinking, and shopping approach. You may also benefit from guidance on cutting out specific food components, particularly fermentable carbohydrates.

Eating more slowly, looking at the FODMAP diet (if symptoms are consistent with Irritable Bowel Syndrome), and considering the use of dietary supplements or a low-GI diet that results in abdominal distension can all help.